Gluten Free, Dairy Free Smoothies & Healing Drinks

Guaranteed to Give You Your Life Back!

by Jaqui Karr, cgp, csn, cvd

Health Coaches, Nutritionists, anyone advising on food or health: get details about my comprehensive Gluten Course for Professionals

It will help you talk gluten at Expert Level *fast* so you can get great results

Go to JaquiKarr.com for details

I put together this cookbook series quite reluctantly (3 in this series: soups/appetizers, dips, drinks/smoothies; and a 4th called "NakedFood" to help people add a little more raw to their existing diets with extra easy fast recipes). I didn't want to do any kind of cookbook at all because I knew I didn't have the time for proper photography, finding graphic designer, editor, etc.

But the #1 question I kept getting at seminars, workshops, and even on social media was "What do you personally eat?"

It seems a lot of people had many 500 page cookbooks, but they were just collecting dust in their kitchen. What's the use of 500 recipes if you never do any of them? You're better off with 15 that you use constantly and keep making variations to (I teach you how to do that so you end up with endless variations).

So without the beauty of a proper setting or professional photographer, I started to simply document everything I personally (ate). I did this on quiet writing days, busy days just before heading to the airport, and even on my quiet Sunday tea-in-bed morning.

I did my best with the pictures. Some turned out great, others "did the job" but made me want to invest in a 3000 dollar camera and studio box.

The end result: recipes of power food I eat and for some really important staple ingredients, I also explain why I eat it. Nothing fancy. Just very practical and simple.

Stay Healthy, Live Well. Life's too short for bad food.

It's not just smoothies...

Throughout the ages there have always been magical elixirs known to heal as well as poison. Nothing has changed.

You can flood your system with sugar, chemicals, and hidden glutens (sadly, mocha isn't just chocolate anymore) or you can choose to make yourself drinks that power you up completely naturally.

Not only can drinks power you up as in give you usable energy to get through your day, but drinks can also:

--boost your immune system

--clear your skin

--purify and alkalize your blood

--satisfy you and keep you from overeating

--keep your blood sugar balance

--help regulate your mood

--provide a full day's worth of vitamins & minerals

--keep you hydrated, making you function optimally

--help prevent disease

--and of course, give you pure pleasure!

And so my gorgeous Gods and Goddesses,
Choose your elixirs wisely and remember that life is meant to be enjoyed. Everything becomes so much more enjoyable when you do it from a strong healthy state.

Jaqui Karr

FIG & CHOCOLATE ELIXIR 7

    RAW CACAO 8

MAYAN COCOA, Drink of the Gods 9

    "EXCITOTOXINS" 10

CHOCO COCO SMOOTHIE 11

THE POWER BLUE TONIC 12

    SPIRULINA 13

HEALING PLUM COCKTAIL 14

PURPLE MAGIC 15

PIÑA BANANA MANGO SMOOTHIE 16

STRESS BUSTING SUNSHINE SMOOTHIE 17

WATERMELON MARTINI 18

WATERMELON & CHERRY 19

CANTALOUPE & CHERRY COOLER 20

FIG & RASPBERRY SMOOTHIE 21

MINT, AN ANCIENT HEALER 22

MOJITO WITH A TWIST 23

GREENS ROCK! 24

CELERY CUKE COCKTAIL 25

COCONUT BLAST 26

TROPICAL BEACH SMOOTHIE 27

    COCONUT WATER 27

RASPBERRY SMOOTHIE 28

    LEFTOVER SMOOTHIE MIX 29

SMOOTH KIWI 30

NOT-SO-PEAR SMOOTHIE 31

AN APPLE A DAY 32

WHEAT GRASS WONDER 33

PROPER HYDRATION 34

WATER INFUSIONS 36

    SAGE 36

    CITRUS 37

TEA TIME 38

CHOCOLATE FEVER

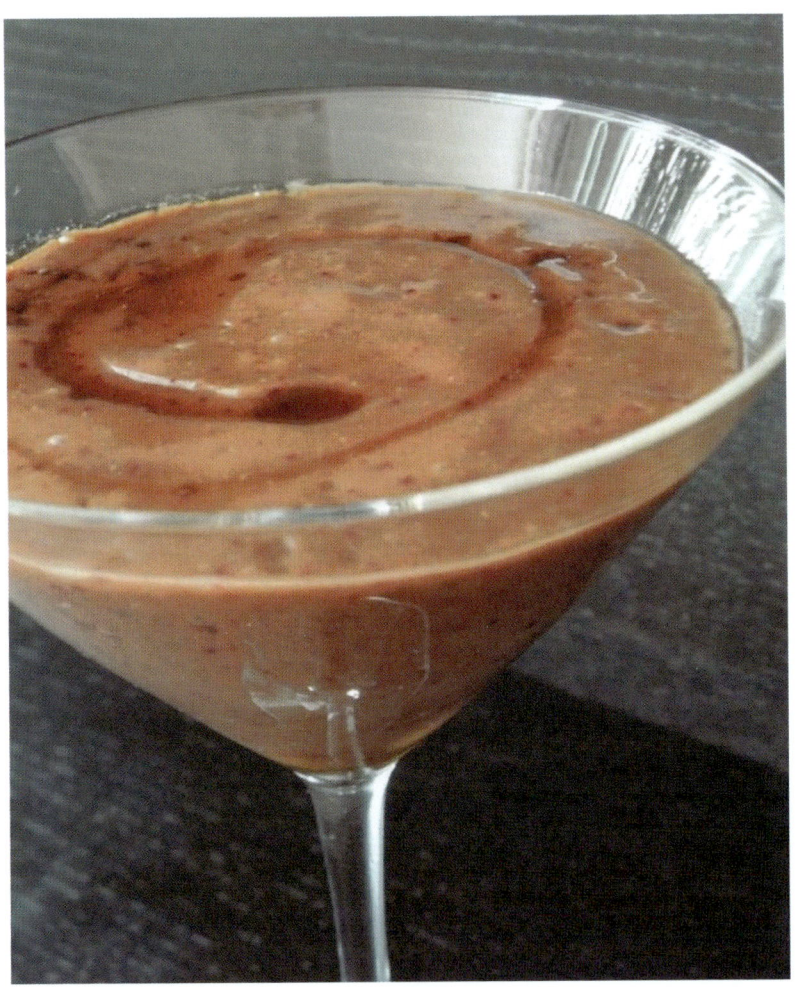

FIG & CHOCOLATE ELIXIR

My secret to maintaining fantastically healthy eating habits is to create foods and beverages that are appetizing, are visually appealing, and incredibly delicious. No will power required – it's a pure joy to eat well!

IN A BLENDER:

½ cup fresh figs

½ cup coconut milk

½ tsp raw cacao

pinch of nutmeg

3 tbsp maple syrup to drizzle

The trick to versatility is sometimes something as simple as what you serve in…

This very drink in a regular glass or travel mug is a delicious start to the day or snack; served in a martini glass it is suddenly an elegant dessert (and perfect for times when you don't have time to actually make dessert)

TIP: use 1 cup of figs instead of ½ cup and it becomes thick enough to be a pudding

RAW CACAO (unprocessed chocolate)

CACAO has become a controversial topic in the nutrition world, with many calling it a stimulant or drug, and addictive *(we kind of all knew that last part)*. But let's have a look…

Beginning at Harvard: Dr. Eric L. Ding says that cocoa potentially prevents heart disease due to its polyphenolic flavonoids. Their 21 studies involved 2575 participants and found associations to healthier cholesterol levels, improved blood vessel health, and decreased blood pressure. Another Harvard study followed 8000 of its own graduates and found the ones who consumed more chocolate lived longer.

Let's backtrack to 1500 B.C. The Mayans called it "chocolatl", literally a sacred drink for the gods to be drunk from golden cups, enhancing health and providing strength. The Mayans weren't alone; The Greek term "theobroma" means "food of the gods", and the cacao comes from the Theobroma tree. The Aztecs believed it had special powers, reserving it for their nobles, priests, and warriors.

Back to modern day: it is one of the most complex foods on earth with over 300 components to it, full of antioxidants and countless incredible properties including 4x the anti-aging compound found in the goji berry. The studies are ongoing and no doubt will continue to be – though I doubt we'll live to see the human mind decipher and understand the complexity of this food that was made for the goddess & god in each of us.

Cacao, cocoa, chocolate,… there is a long list of names because cacao has been around for thousands of years through hundreds of cultures, seeing changes in spelling & pronunciation with each new culture. Whichever name you use, be sure you are using raw organic, unprocessed cacao.

MAYAN COCOA, Drink of the Gods

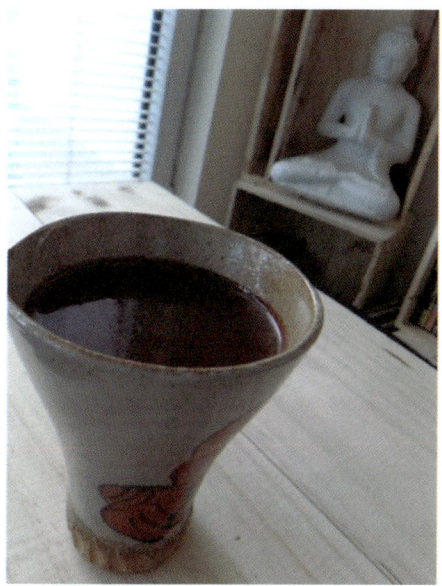

PER CUP (slowly stir with a whisk on low heat)

1 cup almond milk (water)

2 tsp raw cocoa powder

pinch of cayenne pepper

pinch of ground cinnamon

maple syrup if you require sweetening

"EXCITOTOXINS"

I must address the issue some people who react to chocolate and doctors and nutritionists who feel chocolate is bad for you…

Loving cacao as I do, you can imagine I have taken a close look at the matter. The people I have come across who claimed they had issues seemed to have one or both of the problems:

1) They were clearly over-doing it with chocolate, consuming shakes and smoothies with heaping spoons of chocolate several times a day

2) They were not consuming pure organic raw cacao. Anytime you consume a toxic sugar-loaded product, you can expect adverse reactions sooner or later

There may legitimately be people who react to 'the good stuff", but that is true of everything from apples to kale. My personal belief is that with our contaminated food supply and ever increasing number of people with allergies and auto-immune disorders, we are going to find more and more people reacting to more and more foods.

When it comes to ancient foods like cacao, tea (I may as well address the caffeine issue while we are on the topic) – I would be looking more closely at the person's overall state of health and possible underlying issues that have not been discovered or allergies tested for.

CHOCO COCO SMOOTHIE

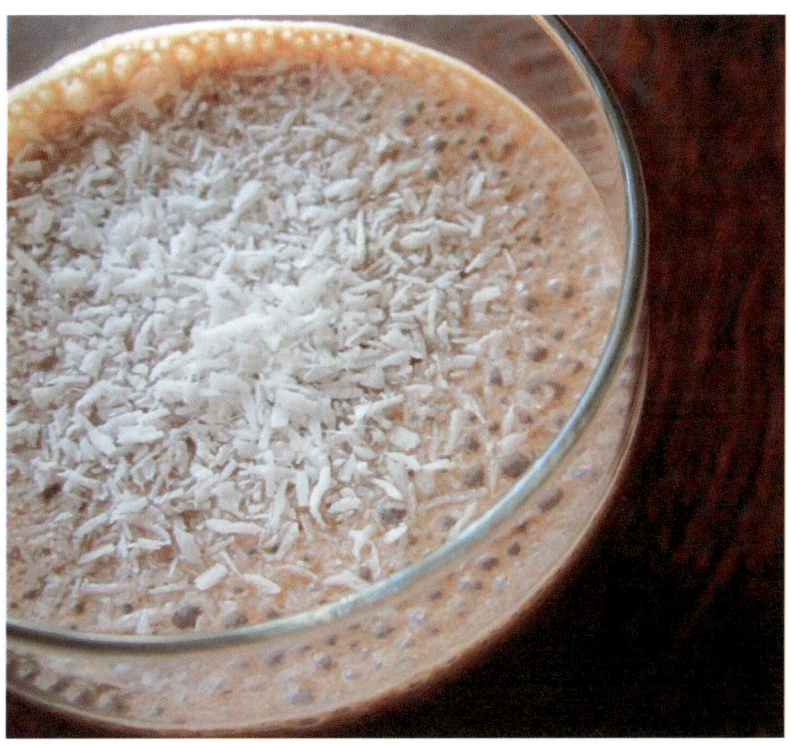

IN THE BLENDER:
1 banana
1 cup coconut water
1 cup almond milk
2 tsp raw cacao
2 tsp shredded coconut
1 tsp ground flax
1oz aloe vera juice (optional, excellent for healing)
3 ice cubes

HEALING AND STRENGTHENING

THE POWER BLUE TONIC

IN THE BLENDER:
1 cup blueberries (or mixed berries)
1 heaping tbsp spirulina
1 tsp raw cacao
1 cup coconut water (or plain water)
1 tbsp organic blackstrap molasses (adds iron)
1 tsp wheat grass powder (certified gluten free)
1 oz aloe vera juice (2 if you are a recovering Celiac)
7-8 walnuts (omega-3's)
3-5 Brazil nuts (organic adds selenium)
OPTIONAL: 3-4 Medjool dates (this adds sweetness, nutrition, and also highly usable raw energy)

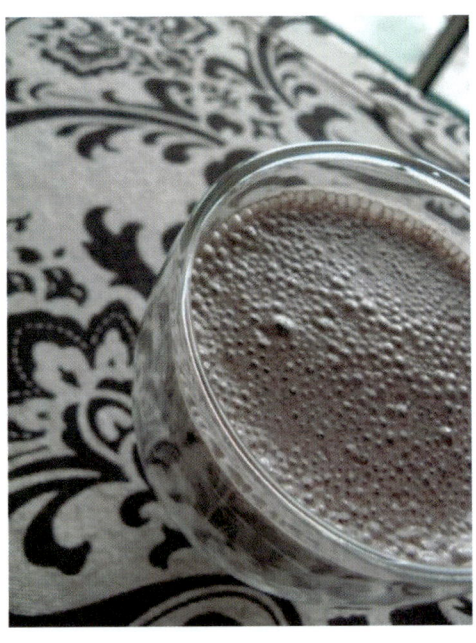

SPIRULINA

I'm asked some questions more often than others: 1) At 40 years old how do you still play racquetball with 20 year old partners back to back AND still have energy left over 2) how did you recover from extensive Celiac damage so quickly 3) why do you never get a cold? (well, I do get a cold... *once a decade*). The answer to all 3 questions is the same: I drink and eat foods that help the body:
1) heal itself and renew cells
2) be armed with an army of nutrients

An absolute miracle food: B_1, B_2, B_3, B_6, B_{12}, C, D, E, K, folic acid, pantothenic acid, biotin, inositol, calcium, magnesium, potassium, phosphorus (is in every cell throughout the body and works with calcium to maintain bone density), chromium, selenium, and a great source for iron (10x higher than normal foods). The phycocyanin in it (blue pigment) combines with iron and other minerals making them more bioavailable (2x more than meats and vegetables).

10g of spirulina provides 23,000 I.U. of beta carotene which the body converts to Vitamin A and unlike taking Vitamin A supplements (fat soluble, too much can be toxic), when it is your body doing the converting, it automatically stops at the right amount - *such a miraculous thing the body is*, in its natural form. **Beta carotene** is a powerful antioxidant that fights free radicals and also reduces the body's risks to several types of cancer including colon and gastrointestinal tract. Spirulina is a complete protein that delivers all essential amino acids in a highly absorbable form, as well as zeaxanthin/lutein which are important for eye health.

HEALING PLUM COCKTAIL

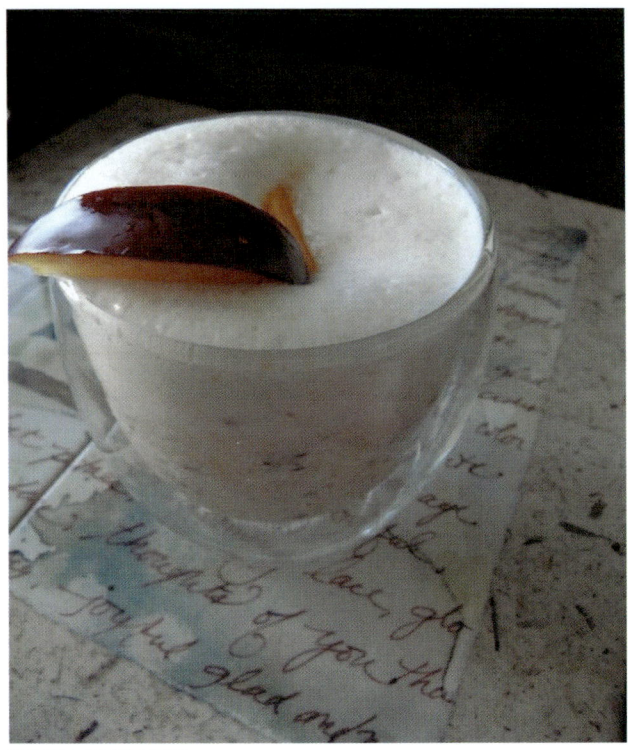

IN BLENDER:
2 plums
1 apricot (or peach)
2 Medjool dates
1 tbsp of organic blackstrap molasses*
2 cups coconut water or coconut milk
½ tspn nutritional yeast (adds B12)
3-4 Brazil nuts (optional, adds selenium, a mineral often deficient for those with Celiac Disease)
(optional) 2oz aloe vera juice
*one tablespoon provides the average person with 20% of their daily iron requirements; just be sure you are getting pure organic blackstrap and not molasses made from corn

PURPLE MAGIC

I personally love the taste of raw cacao and it certainly can be a lifesaver in getting someone to consume spirulina if they don't like the taste of it – though there are enough berries in this recipe to be able to mask the other flavors well on their own. This smoothie is so berrilicious, it's hard to imagine what a powerful cleanser and detoxifier it is!
Cheers, to your health

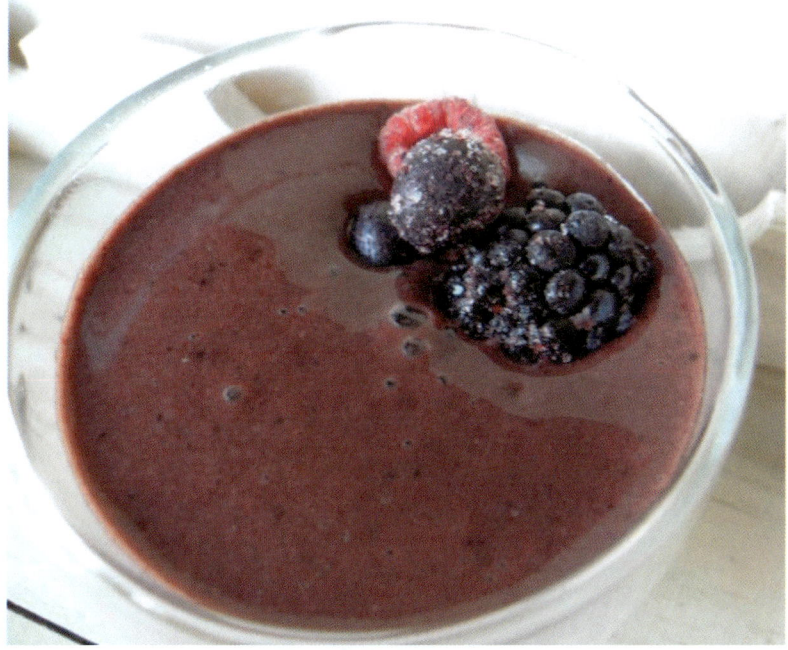

2 cups frozen berries (shown here with equal parts of strawberries, raspberries, blackberries, and blueberries)
1 tbsp liquid chlorophyll
1 tsp spirulina
1 cup water
(optional) 1 tbsp raw cacao
(optional) maple syrup or honey to sweeten

PIÑA BANANA MANGO SMOOTHIE

BLEND: 1 mango, 1 banana, 1 cup coconut milk, and 2 cups pineapple – Can it get any simpler? And SO refreshing! I love serving it with a piece of dehydrated mango, transforms it into dessert!

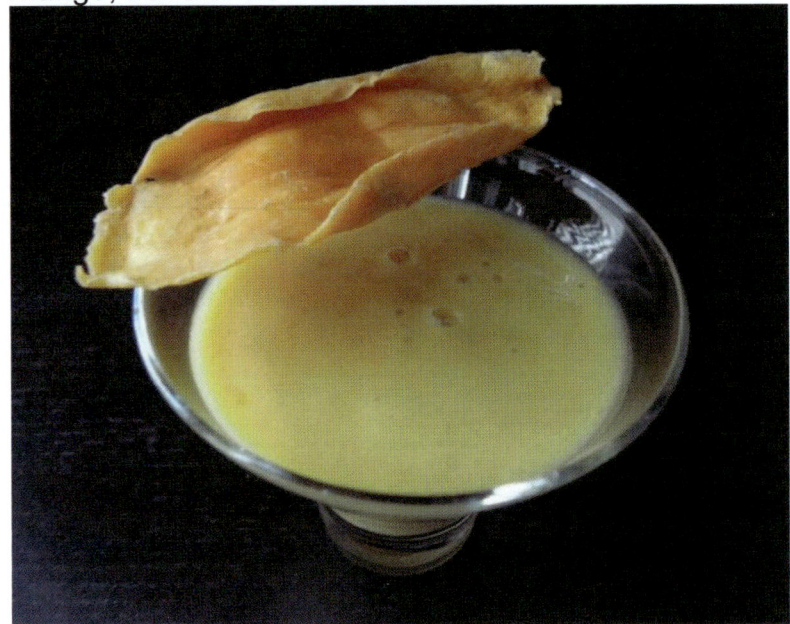

START YOUR DAY OFF RIGHT!

Stress. We all have way too much of it in our lives. Your body has to battle the dreaded chemical flooding of cortisol every time you feel stress… but what are you arming your body to fight it with? Get your blender out and let me tell you how to start your day off with a huge hit of 2 fantastic stress busting vitamins: C and B6.

The Stress-Busting Sunshine Smoothie gives you 210mg (353% of a day's worth) of vitamin C, 1.3mg of B6 (67%), plus 2 extra bonuses 1841 IU of vitamin A (37%) and 15g of fiber (58%).

STRESS BUSTING SUNSHINE SMOOTHIE

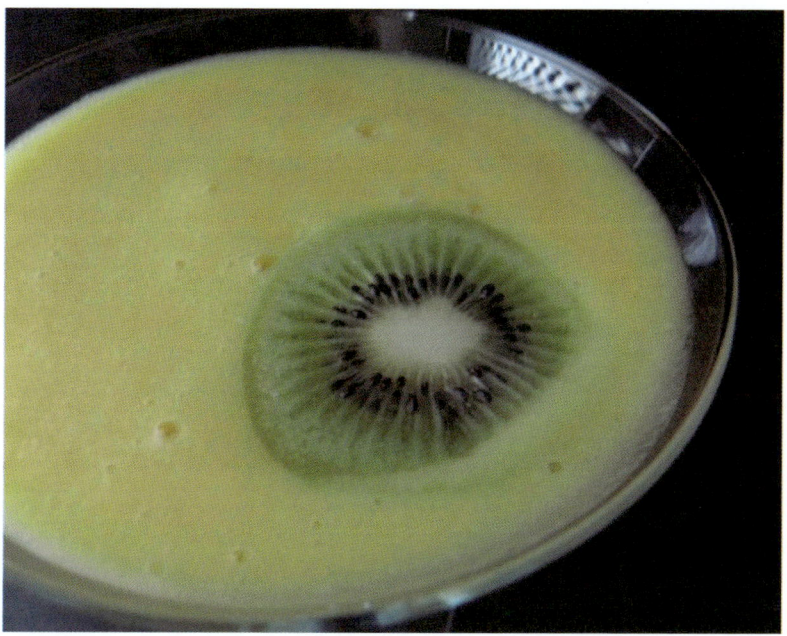

BLEND: 1 cup pineapple, 1 banana, 1 orange, and 1 cup mango (I prefer the "champagne"/yellow variety)

TIP: add 1 more banana to the mix and you bring your B6 intake up to 100%/RDA.

GOOD TO KNOW: the fruit with the LEAST punch in this mix? The orange. Which is surprising to most people since oranges have become synonymous with vitamin C. And that is good news because the other 3 are easy to keep in the freezer and have on hand at all times. So if you didn't have a chance to grocery shop and you skip the orange - it's no problem! Now depending on how much fresh vs. frozen is in your mix, adjust water and ice to your liking to get the thickness you enjoy most.

WATERMELON MARTINI

Ever wonder what to do with those leftover pieces of watermelon from hot summer days? This drink is so special you won't wait for leftovers from Sunday lunches!

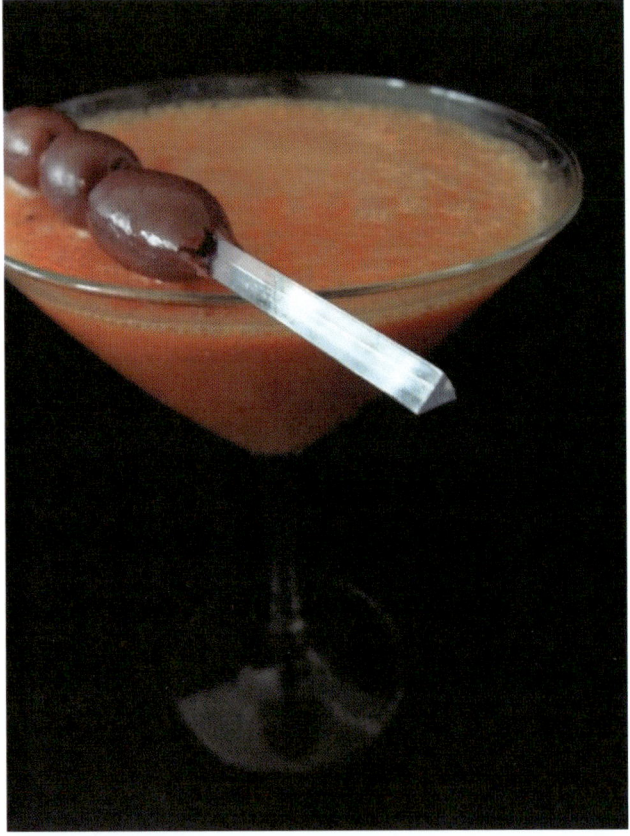

IN BLENDER:
3 cups cold watermelon (or add some ice cubes if it is at room temperature)
3/4 cup sun dried tomatoes
1 tsp cayenne pepper (or paprika)
1 tbsp thyme

WATERMELON & CHERRY

I'll begin with the warning: this is VERY high in fiber (which can be a remedy to certain problems) but also something to be aware of as I wouldn't want to cause discomfort.

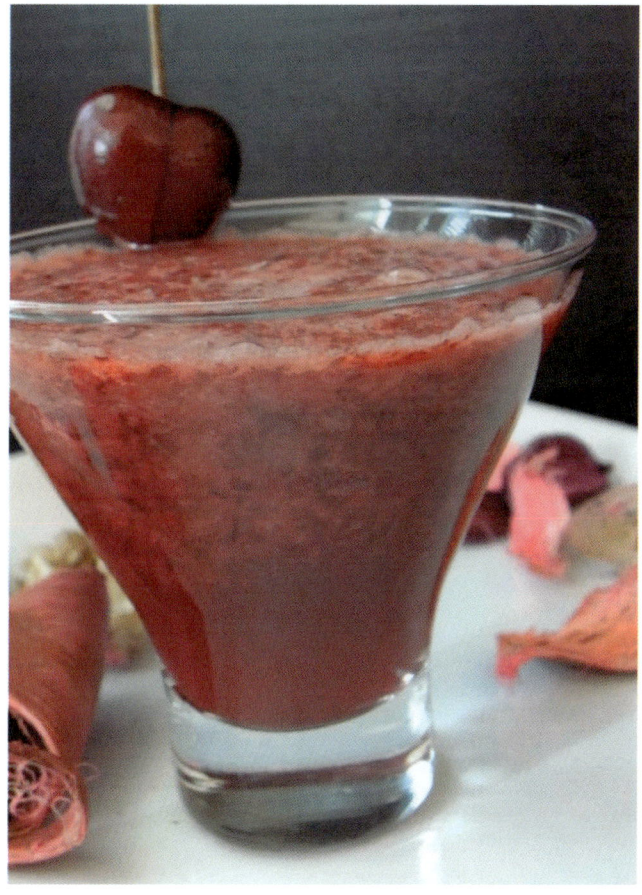

Watermelon and pitted cherries in the blender with some ice and you have a powerful flavor you have never tasted before! This is so rich in flavor, I can't describe!

CANTALOUPE & CHERRY COOLER

Leftovers are the best thing to hit my kitchen! I always end up making something new in an effort to not waste anything. In this case it was slices of cantaloupe leftover from breakfast…

MEASUREMENTS NOT NEEDED

Just toss cantaloupe into the blender (you don't need to add water), blend, and pour into glasses, leaving just a tiny bit in the blender.

ADD TO THAT BIT some pitted cherries and blend again, then spoon that mixture over the cantaloupe. Done. Fun!

Easy, as usual

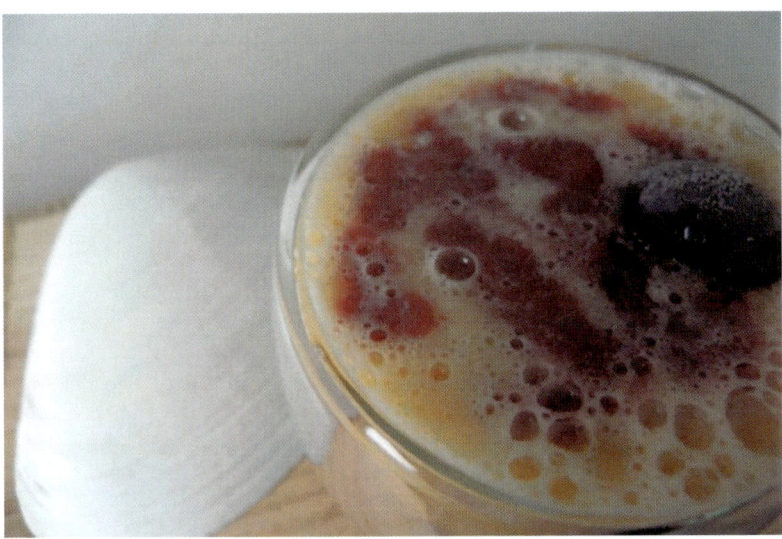

FIG & RASPBERRY SMOOTHIE

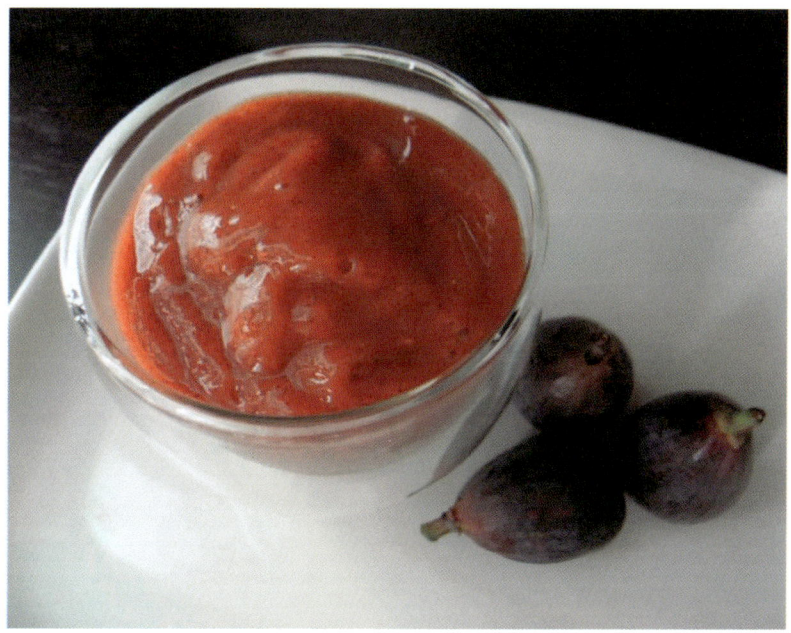

I love figs. I absolutely adore figs. But I live in Canada and this means I have access to figs for a very short period of time at the end of summer… which causes me to buy them by the case. And as much as I love them, once in a while I end up with a whole lot of them that are way too ripe before I've had a chance to eat them.

Smoothie? Sorbet? Yes and yes. Same recipe – you can drink it on the spot or freeze it for later.

BLEND: equal parts figs and raspberries, add water to get desired thickness. Nutrient factor here is sky high!

MINT, AN ANCIENT HEALER

…you'll be pleasantly surprised…

--excellent for anyone with digestive disorders, stomach aches

--has a calming effect, used to help with headaches, depression, & insomnia

--contains menthol, thymol, carvacrol – all fight flatulence

--increases perspiration, thereby decreasing fever

--protects the liver and helps it function more efficiently

--reduces pain for those with gallstones or kidney stones

--antifungal properties are fantastic to help relieve issues in the respiratory tract & asthma issues

--helps with diarrhea and IBS discomfort

--improves blood circulation

--contains perillyl alcohol, an anti-cancer property

--decreases altitude sickness (hikers/climbers, start having infusions from 3-4 days ahead)

--its antioxidants are said to prevent cataracts (though you would need to consume several cups every day to intake enough for this)

--last but not least, it even freshens the breath, so enjoy your minty drinks and make sure you kiss a loved one!

MOJITO WITH A TWIST

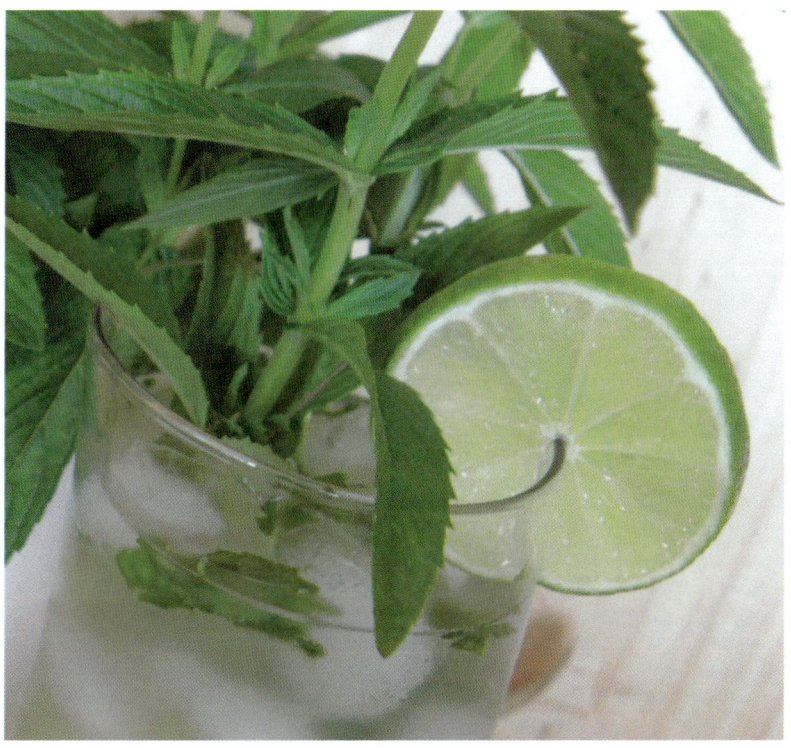

--Crush a handful of mint (mortar & pestle are best, but improvise if you don't have them, you can use a wooden spoon or just chop & smash), along with a small piece of fresh ginger and the juice of ½ a lime

--Put the mixture in a tall glass, add ice & water, and think of something wonderful to toast to!

--VARIATION: try sweet basil instead of mint, it's fantastic!

NOTE: add maple syrup if you'd like some sweetness, do avoid toxic white sugar as most Mojito recipes call for

GREENS ROCK!

Even if you are not the healthiest eater, starting your day with an alkalinizing drink like this will help your body counter toxins. ...that doesn't mean I am endorsing toxic food and that this kind of drink is a ticket to eat poorly, but the reality is most people won't have that perfect, totally pure diet – but by making some very healthy, highly potent additions, they will certainly give their body more to fight with and lower their risks to health issues.

You might notice I am blending and not juicing, which is what most people do with greens. While I do also juice, I think it's great to drink food as a whole sometimes – maintaining fiber and other components that juicing would eliminate.

Greens, more than any other foods, have an amazing ability to heal and strengthen your body. Greens simultaneously detoxify and nourish, while turning back the hands of time to help you look and feel younger.

Regular staples I consume absolutely every week in one form or another:
--broccoli or asparagus
--collard greens (they make the perfect wrap)
--cucumber
--kale
--parsley or coriander
--spinach
--watercress
--wheat grass or spirulina (sea vegetable, but still a vegetable!)

CELERY CUKE COCKTAIL

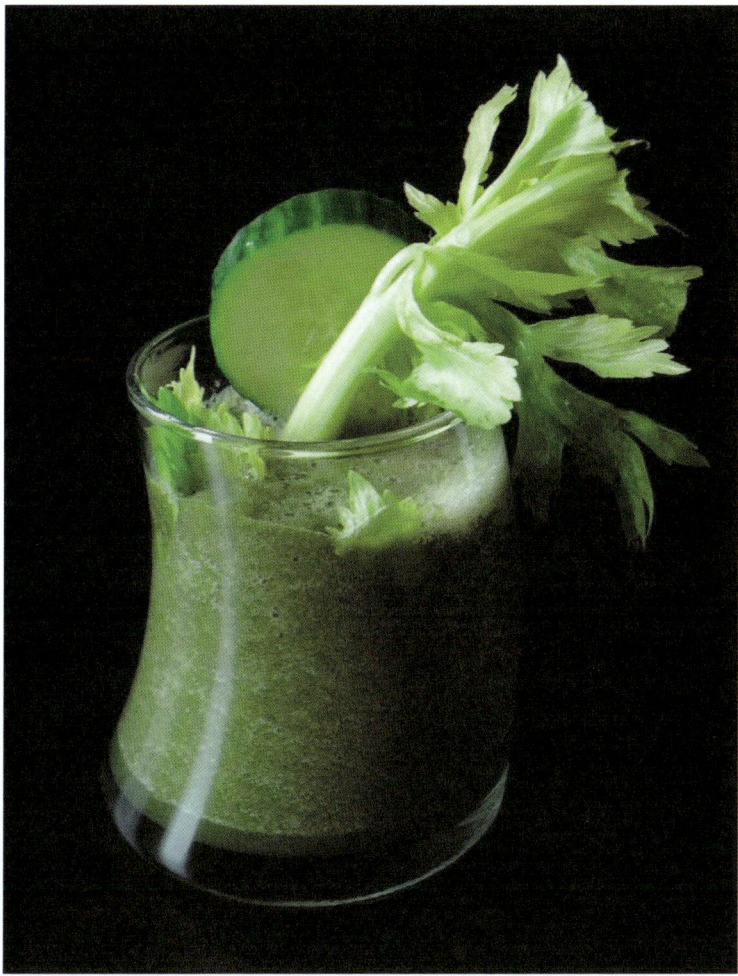

IN BLENDER: 4 stalks celery, 1 cup cucumber (with peel), 1 tbsp wheat grass powder, 2 cups coconut water

TIP: do not peel the cucumber, the skin has anti-aging properties! Just make sure you are buying organic

REFRESH, REJUVENATE, AND TURN BACK TIME!

COCONUT BLAST

2 cups coconut meat
1 cup coconut water
½ frozen ripe banana
1 cup fresh or frozen pineapple
Served with dehydrated coconut flakes

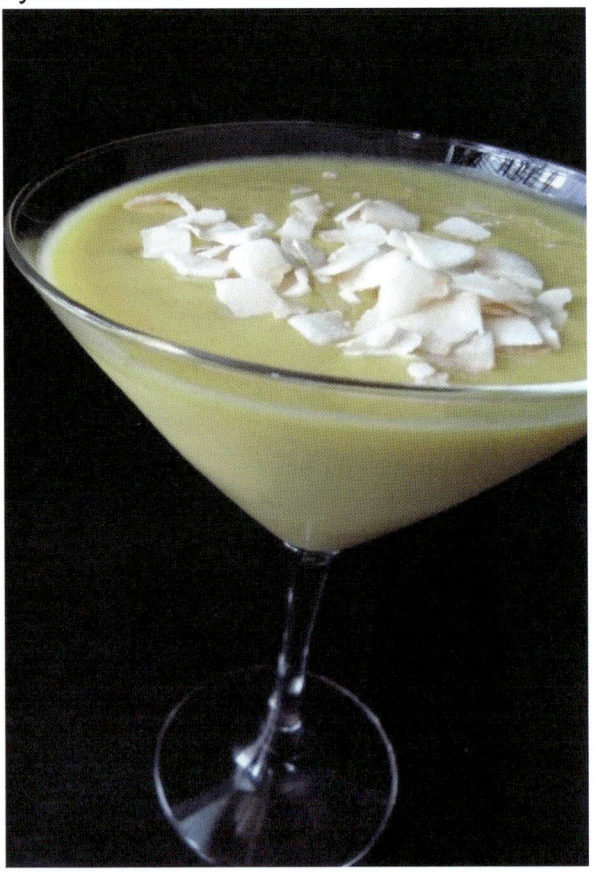

TROPICAL BEACH SMOOTHIE

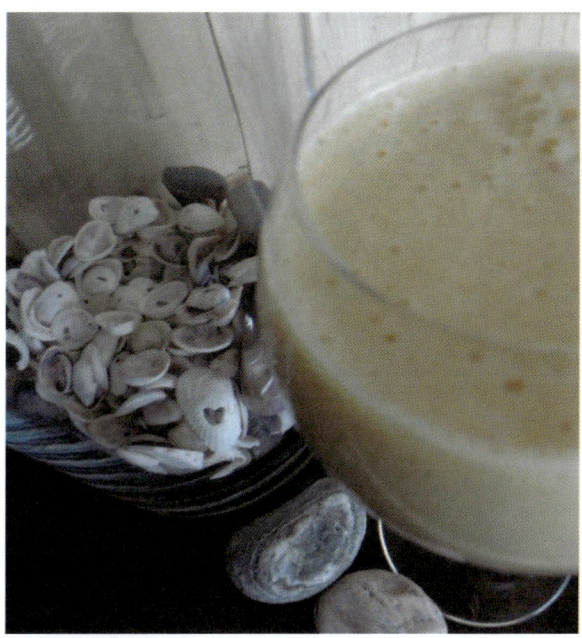

IN BLENDER:
1 banana
1 apricot or peach
½ cup pineapple (fresh or frozen)
½ cup frozen mango or papaya
2 cups coconut water or coconut milk, or 1 cup coconut water and 1 cup freshly squeezed orange juice

COCONUT WATER bursting with electrolytes and potassium, it carries oxygen and nutrients to your cells, regulates body temperature, helps balance pH levels, hydrates, detoxifies, and has amazing anti-viral, anti-fungal, and anti-microbial properties that not only prevent disease but have been known to help cure many diseases. And the taste is heavenly!

RASPBERRY SMOOTHIE

All too often I see people over complicating what is actually simple. In a mad rush to "power up" and get lots of nutrition and antioxidants and the long list of vitamins we are being scared into consuming every day, people are making these huge smoothies containing a dozen ingredients, mixing greens, fruit, supplements, you name it! I don't even know if our bodies are designed to efficiently absorb that much all at the same time. Keep it simple: we know antioxidants are great, we know all berries have them, whatever you find in organic form or have in your freezer – blend it up and you're good to go. Keeping it simple will also allow you to appreciate every flavor.

BLENDER:
1 cup frozen or fresh raspberries
1 cup cantaloupe
½ cup water
Add ice if you want a thicker colder "smoothie" texture

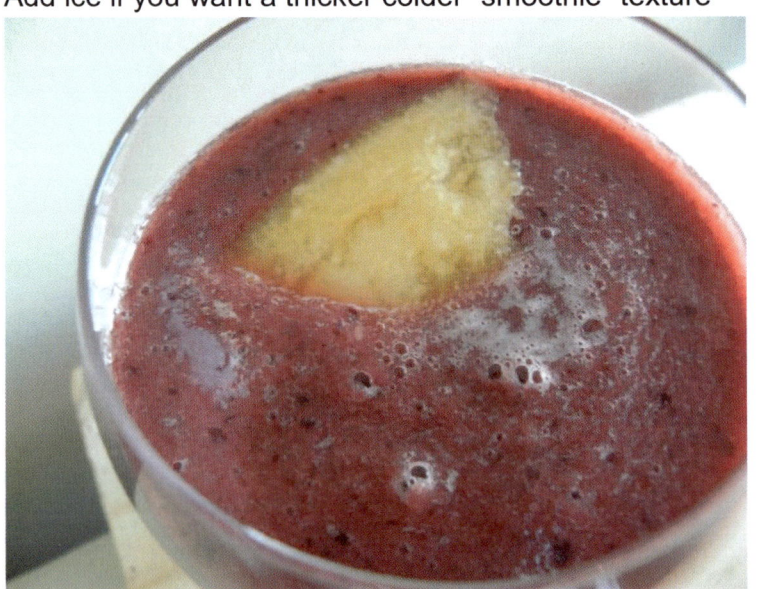

LEFTOVER SMOOTHIE MIX

…hold on to that mix and get your ice cube tray or dessert molds! That leftover mix is golden! Not only do you not waste, your freezer will become a treasure chest of ready made desserts (sorbet extraordinaire!) or you might punch up a smoothie that's lacking punch on another day.

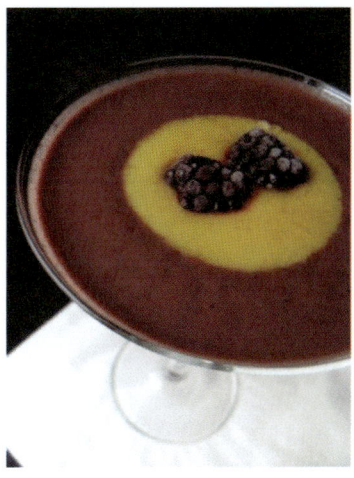

Leftover here is mango, pineapple, banana, coconut water

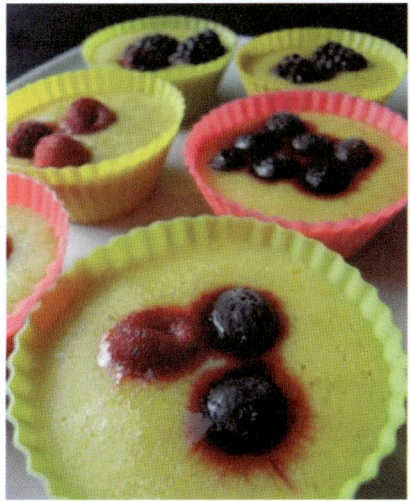

SMOOTH KIWI

KIWIFRUIT I love both the green and golden variety – which have very different tastes. Kiwi are fantastic fruit in terms of nutrition, but please let me say that all plant food is valuable; I don't believe in a diet that focuses on just supposed "super foods" and ignores everything else, so do eat any plant food you can get your hands on and vary as much as possible.

I say "smooth kiwi" instead of calling it a "kiwi smoothie" because the texture of kiwis always make blended drinks so *smoooooottttthhhhhh!* Mixing flavors is always a question of personal taste, so experiment to see what you like, but kiwi is a fruit I myself don't seem to like mixing with a whole lot of other fruits. The ones I do enjoy mixing kiwi with: banana, pineapple, coconut. My usual mix is kiwi, banana, and coconut milk – simple and refreshing.

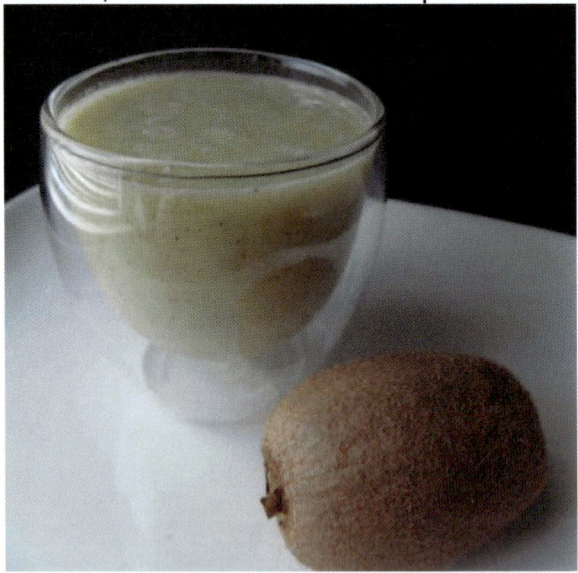

BLENDER: 2 kiwifruit, 2 cups pineapple, 1 cup ice, 1 cup hemp milk (or coconut, or almond)   Optional: ½ banana (I always keep frozen on hand for these)

NOT-SO-PEAR SMOOTHIE

Believe it or not there's a fruit I don't like: pears *(even a vegetable, but we'll leave that for another discussion)*

But I am a firm believer in eating as much from the plant world as I can get my hands on. Every fruit has its own unique combination of nutrients and practicing what I teach I find enjoyable ways to have the ones I'm not that crazy about. "Masking flavors" is easy and worthwhile.

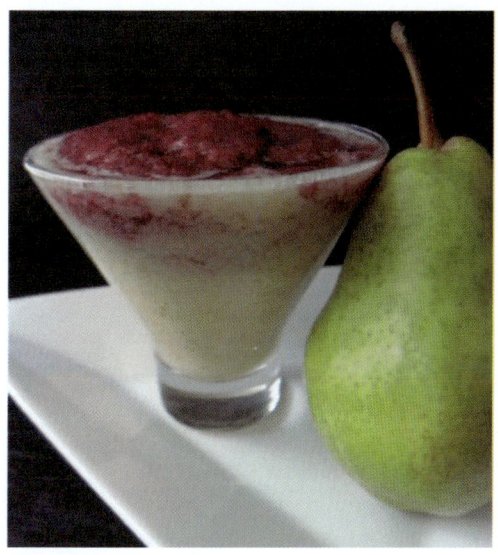

MY NOT-SO-PEAR-TASTING RECIPE:
1-2 dates (more for added sweetness)
1 pear
1/4 tsp cardamom
1/2 cup ice
1/2 cup frozen pineapple
1/2 cup water
--Blend everything and pour half of it into a glass
--Then add 1/2 cup frozen berries (shown here with blueberries, can be any berry) and pour over top

AN APPLE A DAY

Having trouble getting in an apple a day? No trouble!
…toss it into a sinful chocolate berry smoothie and you'll never know it was there!

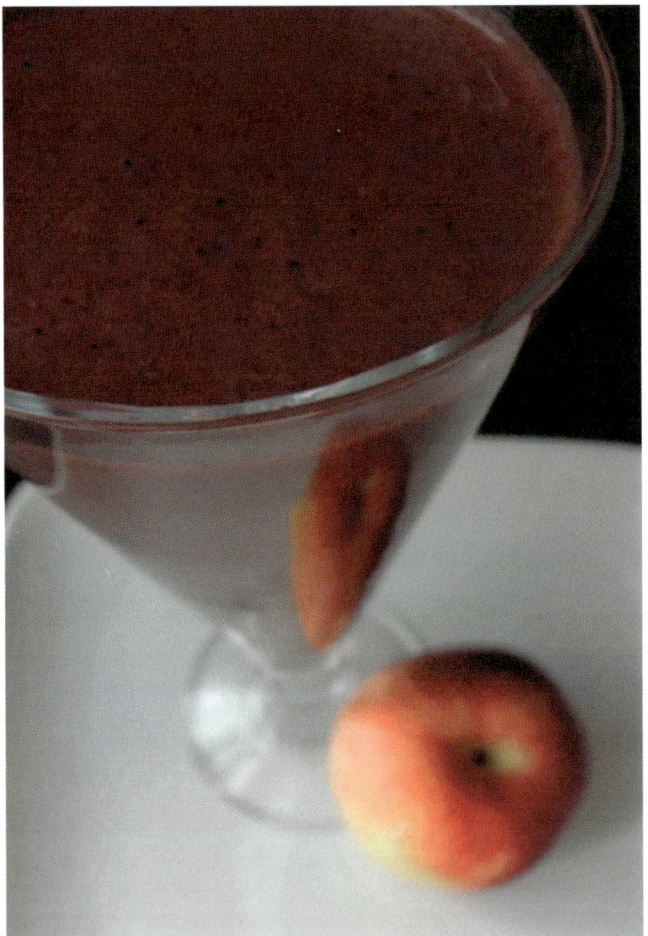

BLEND: 2 cups mixed frozen berries (raspberries, blackberries, blueberries, strawberries), 1 (cored) apple, 2 tsps raw cacao, 1 frozen ripe banana, 2 cups coconut water. Optional: 1 tsp liquid chlorophyll

WHEAT GRASS WONDER

We all know the amazing benefits of wheat grass, though I don't meet a lot of people who like the taste of it. If that's you, here's a great mix for you!

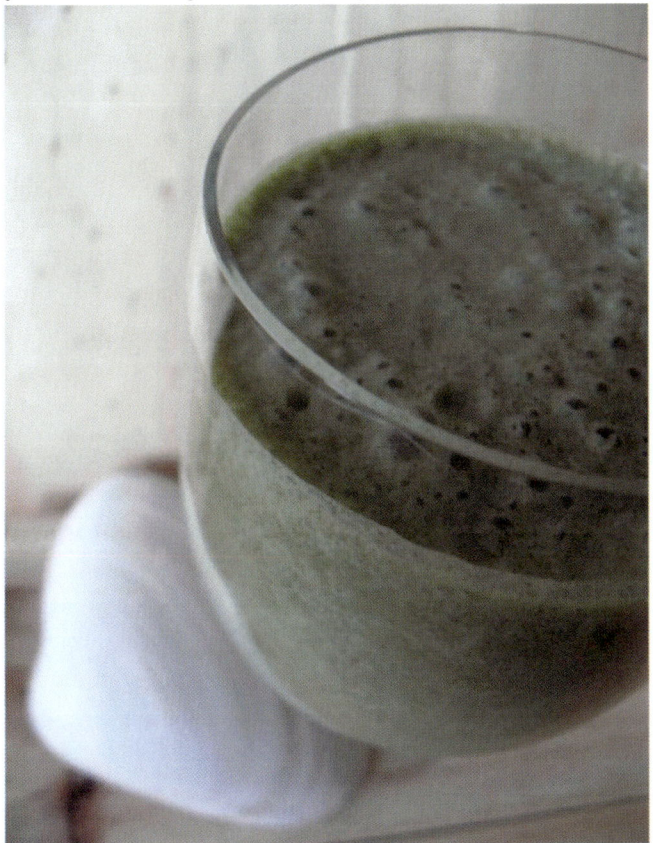

BLEND: 1 frozen banana, ¾ cup water or coconut water ½ cup almond milk, 2 heaping tbsp coconut flakes or coconut meat, 1 heaping tbsp wheat grass powder
GLUTEN ALERT: Wheat GRASS is gluten free, but the seeds are not so make sure you are cutting 1cm away from the seeds or buy certified GF powder as I have here

PROPER HYDRATION

We tend to pay attention to food and track down recipes, cookbooks, even venture out to order exotic ingredients online when we can't find them locally, but the thing we consume that should have priority for our attention is pure clean water.

It is impossible to discuss health & nutrition without mentioning it. Your body needs water to function properly and even if you are 100% raw and eating foods with a high water content, be sure you are still drinking plenty of pure clean water. This is the same for teas (even herbal ones), water infusions, juice,… nothing takes the place of just water.

You'll find it easier to drink more water if it is presented in an appealing way. The beautiful carafe in this photo, along with a tiny burst of color on a tray greets me every morning. I have a tall glass of water before even getting out of bed.

Then throughout the day I have a gorgeous wine goblet on my desk along with a pitcher of water. I am always sure to finish the pitcher. And notice I say "goblet" and not glass. That is because a typical water glass can get very boring. But a beautiful crystal wine goblet or an interesting ceramic tumbler that I found while on a treasure-hunting shopping spree makes the entire experience much more enjoyable; thereby making it an easy habit to maintain.

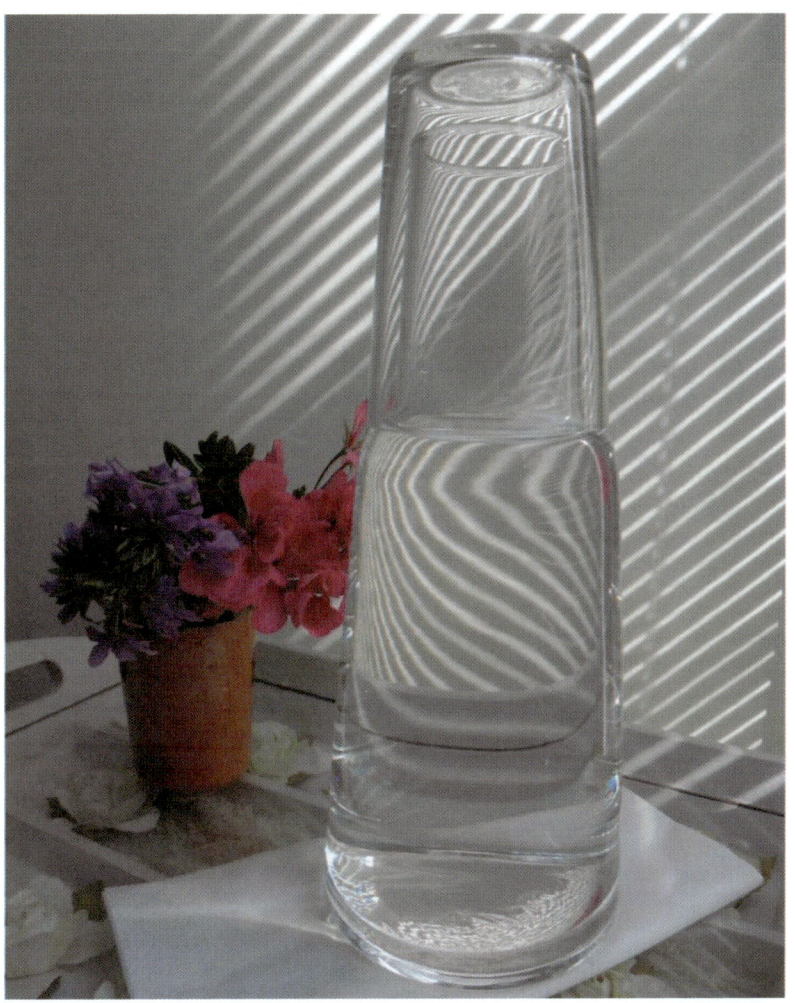

This terrific habit doesn't change when I am out of office or traveling; I bring along a tall stainless steel container no matter where I go. Hydration is the most important word in nutrition; please do take that care of yourself.

WATER INFUSIONS

Always remembering that plain pure water is very important for optimal body function, enjoying flavored water in addition to that is fun and often even has healing properties, as we will examine with sage. As with food, enjoyment and appeal are important, so take the time, find gorgeous containers, and enjoy.

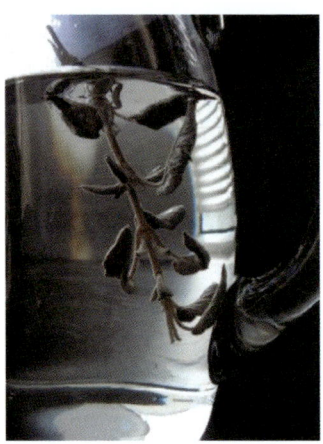

SAGE is an ancient herb used to treat indigestion, depression, female sterility, even menopausal symptoms. It has properties that relax muscle spasms, boost liver function, and reduce feelings of anxiety. If you ever wondered why the lovely scent immediately made you feel at ease, you weren't imagining things!

It is a powerful herb, so don't overdo it, more isn't better in this case; 2-3 glasses a day is fine, I enjoy more sometimes, but take it slow and monitor how you feel.

WARNING: COMPLETELY AVOID SAGE IF PREGNANT, it may act as an abortifacient due to high levels of a component called thujone

CITRUS

Whether it be lemon, lime, orange, or grapefruit as I have here, citrus make delicious infusions.

We generally cut the fruit and thrown slices into the water; what we ignore is the peel, which is bursting with flavor and so easy to store for use anytime.

The next time you are about to eat a fruit or squeeze lemon onto your salad, cut out the peel of the entire fruit in spirals and just leave on the counter (or in the sun) to dry. Once completely dried you can store these in a glass jar, ready to use for tea or water infusions anytime.

...goes without say... it has to be organic fruit & herbs, otherwise you are just getting toxic chemical infusions.

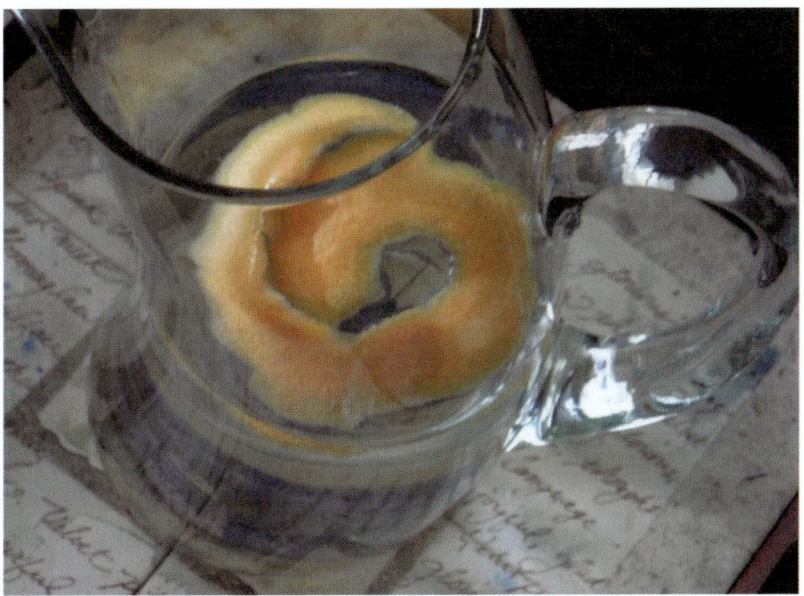

TEA TIME

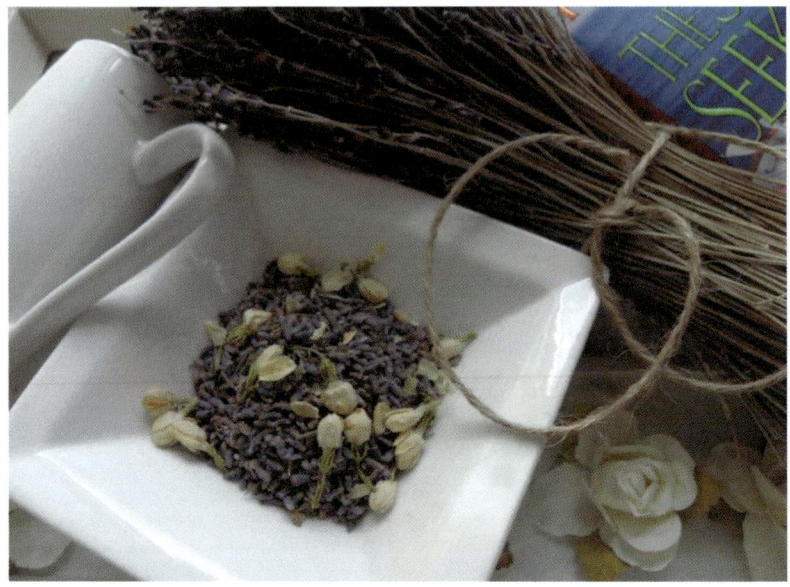

It is technically easy to talk about the wonderful properties of many teas: cinnamon & cloves are both strong anti-inflammatories, roses are said to enhance beauty and be wonderful for the complexion, lavender is calming…

But the element we often forget is the healing quality of just taking the time out to have tea. I have made it a ritual in my life to devote my Sunday mornings to bringing a tea tray to bed and reading for my own leisure. In my field of work, I am constantly reading studies and books that add to my knowledge base, constantly doing research, leaving no time for the fiction books I love – so I make time. That time is mine, it is when I am completely relaxed, the wonderful aroma of whatever tea I have chosen that day is soothing and although I cannot technically measure it, I know that this precious time contributes so much to my overall well being. *I love tea time.*

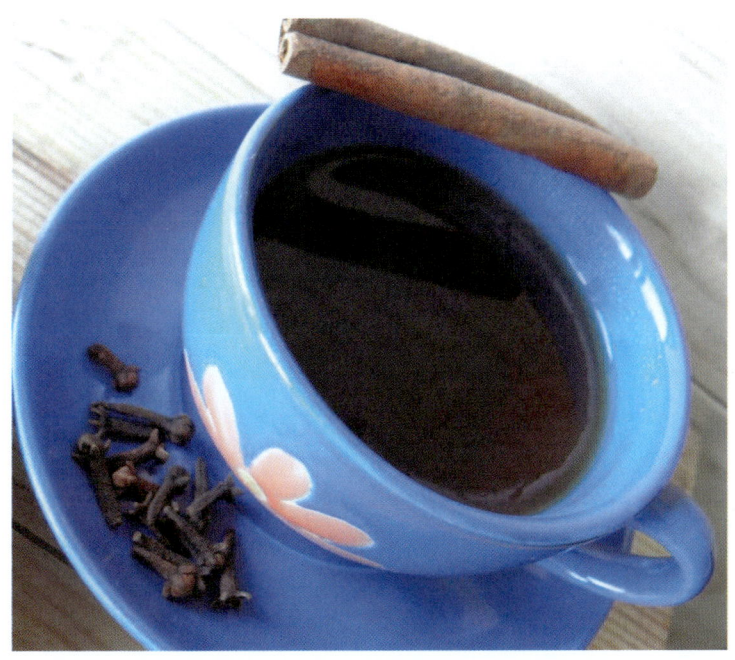

Shown here are lavender & jasmine, cinnamon & cloves, white tea & dried roses. *Always take time out for yourself!*

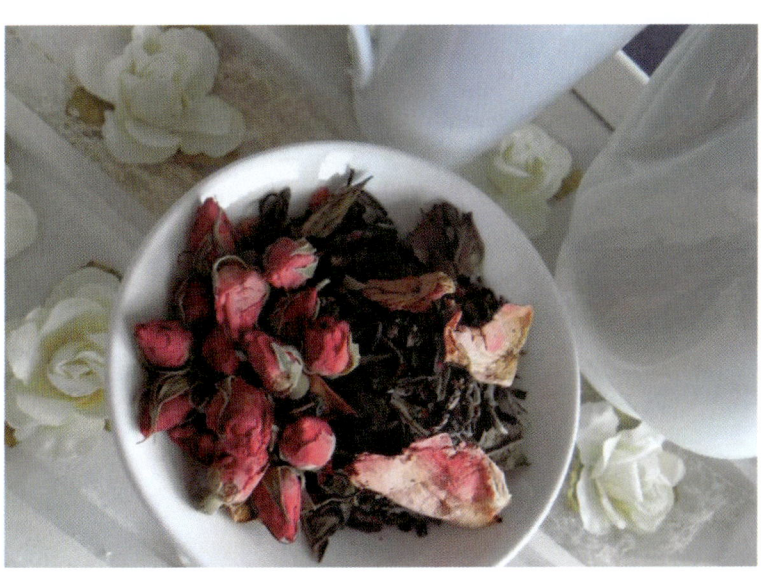

Copyright © 2012 Black Wave Publishing

All rights reserved. Reproduction in any manner without written permission is prohibited except for brief quotations for review or media purposes.

Library and Archives Canada

Author: Karr, Jaqui

Title: Gluten Free, Dairy Free, Sugar Free Smoothies & Healing Drinks Guaranteed to Give You Your Life Back!

ISBN: 978-0-9869039-5-3

Publication Date: April 13, 2012

This book should not be used for diagnosing or treating medical issues. Always consult a trained medical professional with regards to health problems.

Printed in Great Britain
by Amazon